NATURAL HEALING BIBLE FOR BEGINNERS

[6 in 1] The Ultimate Guide to Herbal Remedies, Essential Oils, Infusions, Tinctures, and Antibiotics - Cultivate and Utilize Healing Herbs for Optimal Wellness and Liveliness.

Andrew L. Pabon

TABLE OF CONTENTS

INTRODUCTION

Welcome to Natural Healing Bible for Beginners: [7 in 1], a thoughtful and comprehensive guide designed to help you embark on a journey toward natural wellness and vitality. In our fast-paced world, where synthetic solutions often take center stage, there is a growing desire to reconnect with the ancient wisdom of natural healing. This book is your gateway to understanding and applying time-honored remedies that can transform your approach to health.

Our guide is meticulously crafted to introduce you to the rich world of herbal medicine, essential oils, infusions, tinctures, and natural antibiotics. We start by exploring the basics of herbal remedies, offering a step-by-step approach to cultivating and using healing herbs in your daily life. From growing your own herb garden to preparing simple yet effective herbal treatments, this book equips you with practical knowledge that you can easily integrate into your routine.

Essential oils, another cornerstone of natural healing, are covered in detail. You'll learn about the various oils and their therapeutic properties, how to use them safely and effectively, and how they can complement other natural remedies. Essential oils have been used for centuries to address a range of issues from stress and anxiety to skin care and immune support. With our guidance, you can harness their potent benefits to enhance your overall well-being.

Infusions and tinctures are also integral parts of the natural healing process. We provide clear instructions on how to make these powerful preparations at home, enabling you to create personalized remedies that suit your specific needs. Infusions, made by steeping herbs in hot water, and tinctures, created by extracting herbs in alcohol or vinegar, offer versatile solutions for various health concerns. Our guide simplifies these processes, ensuring that even beginners can confidently craft these beneficial concoctions.

In addition to herbal remedies and essential oils, this book explores the concept of natural antibiotics. While the modern medical world often relies on synthetic antibiotics, nature provides its own powerful alternatives. We delve into the herbs and natural substances that possess antibiotic properties, helping you understand how they can support your body's natural defenses and promote healing.

Throughout this guide, our aim is to make the world of natural healing approachable and actionable. We understand that starting with herbal and holistic remedies can be overwhelming, which is why we've structured this book to build your knowledge gradually. Each section is designed to provide you with a solid foundation, ensuring that you feel confident and informed as you begin to explore and utilize these natural treatments.

By embracing the practices outlined in this book, you're not only learning to address specific health issues but also adopting a holistic approach to wellness. Natural healing is not just about treating symptoms; it's about nurturing your body and mind to achieve a balanced, vibrant life. Whether you're looking to reduce stress, enhance your immune system, or simply explore a more natural way of living, this guide offers the tools and insights you need.

We invite you to delve into the pages of *Natural Healing Bible for Beginners* and discover the power of nature's remedies. As you cultivate and utilize healing herbs, essential oils, infusions, tinctures, and natural antibiotics, you'll uncover a wealth of knowledge that empowers you to take control of your health. Join us on this journey toward a more holistic and fulfilling approach to wellness, and let the natural world be your guide to a healthier, more vibrant life.

BOOK 1: HERBAL APOTHECARY

Chapter 1

How Does Medicinal Plant Work?

Understanding how medicinal plants work involves exploring the fascinating interplay between nature's chemistry and our body's physiology. Medicinal plants have been used for centuries to treat various ailments, and their efficacy lies in the complex compounds they contain, which interact with our body's systems in unique ways.

When you use a medicinal plant, you're essentially introducing a mixture of bioactive compounds into your body. These compounds include alkaloids, flavonoids, terpenes, and glycosides, each with specific effects. For instance, alkaloids such as morphine from the opium poppy have powerful pain-relieving properties, while flavonoids, found in herbs like ginkgo biloba, contribute to antioxidant and anti-inflammatory actions.

Once consumed or applied, these compounds interact with our body at a molecular level. For example, some compounds may bind to receptors in the brain, altering neurotransmitter activity and thereby affecting mood or pain perception. Others might influence the body's inflammatory response, helping to reduce symptoms of conditions like arthritis or asthma. The way these compounds work can vary significantly depending on the plant and the condition being treated.

Moreover, the method of preparation—whether it's a tea, tincture, or topical application—can affect how effectively these compounds are absorbed and utilized by the body. Herbal teas might offer a gentler, more gradual release of their active components, while tinctures, which are more concentrated, can provide a stronger and more immediate effect.

It's also important to consider that medicinal plants often work synergistically. This means that the combined effects of various compounds in the plant can produce a therapeutic outcome that's greater than the sum of its parts. For instance, the combination of different constituents in turmeric—such as curcumin, which has anti-inflammatory properties—works alongside other compounds to enhance its overall healing effect.

Understanding the nuances of how these plants operate can help in making informed choices about their use. It involves appreciating not only the specific actions of individual compounds but also how they interact with each other and with your body. By delving into the world of medicinal plants, you tap into an ancient tradition of healing that is deeply intertwined with the natural world, offering a holistic approach to maintaining health and well-being.

Chapter 2

Foundations of Herbal Remedies and Natural Healing

The foundations of herbal remedies and natural healing are deeply rooted in the rich tapestry of human history, where plants have long been celebrated for their medicinal properties. Understanding these foundations begins with recognizing the intrinsic connection between humans and the natural world, a bond that has guided our use of herbs for thousands of years.

At the heart of herbal remedies is the concept that plants possess unique chemical compounds capable of interacting with our bodies in beneficial ways. These compounds, including essential oils, alkaloids, and flavonoids, have specific actions that can help alleviate symptoms, support health, and promote overall well-being. For instance, the soothing properties of chamomile are attributed to its volatile oils and flavonoids, which work together to calm the digestive system and ease anxiety.

Natural healing also emphasizes the importance of balance and harmony within the body. Unlike conventional medicine, which often targets specific symptoms with isolated treatments, herbal remedies aim to support the body's natural ability to heal itself. This holistic approach considers the interconnectedness of physical, emotional, and spiritual health, recognizing that true wellness involves nurturing all aspects of one's being.

Growing and preparing your own herbs can be an empowering way to connect with these healing traditions. Cultivating herbs in your garden allows you to engage directly with the plants, from sowing seeds to harvesting and using them in remedies. This hands-on approach fosters a deeper understanding of the plants and their properties, enhancing your ability to use them effectively.

Additionally, traditional herbal practices often involve a wealth of knowledge passed down through generations. This knowledge includes not just the

"

physical effects of herbs but also the cultural and historical contexts in which they have been used. Each plant carries its own story, shaped by the experiences of those who have used it for centuries.

Exploring herbal remedies and natural healing is more than just a practice of using plants for health; it's a journey into the wisdom of the natural world. By learning about the properties of different herbs and how they can be used to support your health, you tap into a tradition that values harmony, balance, and the body's inherent ability to heal. This approach encourages a respectful and mindful relationship with nature, honoring the plants that have been our allies in health for millennia.

BOOK 2: HERBS TO KNOW (ABOUT THE HERB, USES AND APPLICATIONS)

Chapter 3

Herbs for Digestive Health

Herbs have long been cherished for their ability to support digestive health, offering natural remedies that address a range of digestive issues. Many cultures have relied on the healing properties of herbs to soothe the digestive system, and their benefits are increasingly recognized in contemporary wellness practices.

Peppermint

One of the most well-known herbs for digestive health is peppermint. Its soothing properties come from menthol, which relaxes the muscles of the gastrointestinal tract and can help alleviate symptoms of irritable bowel syndrome (IBS) and indigestion. Peppermint tea or oil capsules can provide relief from bloating and gas, making it a staple for those seeking natural comfort.

Ginger

Ginger is another powerful herb celebrated for its digestive benefits. Often used to combat nausea, ginger also supports overall digestive function by stimulating saliva, bile, and gastric enzymes. This can improve digestion and reduce feelings of discomfort after eating. Fresh ginger can be added to teas or meals, while ginger supplements are also available for more concentrated effects.

Chamomile

Chamomile, widely known for its calming effects, extends its benefits to digestive health as well. Chamomile tea is a gentle remedy for soothing an upset stomach and reducing inflammation within the digestive tract. Its mild antispasmodic properties can ease digestive cramps and promote relaxation, making it a comforting choice before bedtime.

Fennel seeds

Fennel seeds are another valuable herb for digestive support. They are often used to alleviate bloating and gas, as they help relax the muscles in the gastrointestinal tract and stimulate digestion. Chewing fennel seeds after meals or brewing them into a tea can aid in digestion and reduce discomfort.

Dandelion

Dandelion is a herb that supports liver function and promotes healthy digestion by acting as a gentle diuretic and digestive tonic. It encourages the flow of bile, which is crucial for digesting fats and improving overall digestive efficiency. Dandelion leaves can be used in salads, while the root can be brewed into a tea.

Integrating these herbs into your daily routine can offer a natural approach to maintaining digestive health. Each herb contributes its own unique benefits, and when used thoughtfully, they can complement one another to support a well-functioning digestive system. Embracing these herbal allies invites a holistic approach to digestive wellness, rooted in tradition and supported by nature.

Chapter 4

Herbs for Skin Care

Herbs have long been cherished for their therapeutic benefits, and their use in skin care is no exception. Nature offers a treasure trove of botanical wonders that can help rejuvenate, soothe, and protect the skin.

Chamomile

One of the most revered herbs for skin care is chamomile. Known for its calming properties, chamomile is often used to alleviate skin irritations such as eczema and dermatitis. Its anti-inflammatory and antioxidant properties help to reduce redness and inflammation, while promoting a healthier complexion. Chamomile can be applied topically as a soothing tea or incorporated into creams and lotions to harness its gentle effects.

Calendula

Another powerful herb is calendula, which boasts remarkable healing abilities. Calendula's anti-inflammatory and antimicrobial properties make it an excellent choice for treating cuts, bruises, and minor burns. It also aids in reducing acne and soothing sunburns. Its versatility allows it to be used in various forms, including infusions, salves, and oils, offering a natural remedy for a range of skin issues.

Lavender

Lavender is yet another herb that has earned its place in the realm of skin care. Its calming aroma is matched by its therapeutic benefits. Lavender essential oil is renowned for its ability to balance oily skin and combat acne due to its antimicrobial properties. Additionally, its soothing effects can help alleviate skin irritation and promote relaxation.

Tea tree oil

Tea tree oil, derived from the leaves of the Australian tea tree, is celebrated for its potent antiseptic and anti-inflammatory qualities. It is especially effective in treating acne and fungal infections. When used properly, tea tree oil can help clear up blemishes and improve overall skin clarity.

Aloe Vera

Lastly, aloe vera stands out as a skin-care staple due to its remarkable healing and hydrating properties. Aloe vera gel, extracted from the plant's leaves, can provide relief for sunburns, dry skin, and minor cuts. Its natural soothing agents help to moisturize and repair the skin, making it a popular choice for a variety of skin care routines.

Integrating these herbs into your skin care regimen can offer a natural and effective approach to maintaining healthy skin. Their diverse proportion and applications make them valuable allies in achieving a radiant and balanced complexion.

Chapter 5

Herbs for Emotional Well Being

Herbs have long been valued not only for their physical benefits but also for their profound effects on emotional well-being. These natural remedies offer a gentle yet powerful means of nurturing mental and emotional health.

Lavender

One of the most celebrated herbs for emotional support is lavender. Known for its calming properties, lavender has been used for centuries to reduce stress and anxiety. The soothing scent of lavender can help to calm a restless mind and promote a sense of relaxation. It's often used in aromatherapy, where its essential oil is diffused into the air, or applied topically to help ease tension and improve sleep quality.

Chamomile

Another herb with significant emotional benefits is chamomile. Often consumed as a tea, chamomile is renowned for its mild sedative effects. Drinking chamomile tea before bedtime can help ease anxiety and promote a restful night's sleep. Its gentle nature makes it an ideal choice for those looking for a natural remedy to manage everyday stress and anxiety.

St. John's Wort

St. John's Wort is another powerful herb known for its mood-enhancing properties. This herb has been studied extensively for its potential to alleviate symptoms of depression. By influencing neurotransmitters in the brain, St. John's Wort can help to lift mood and improve emotional balance. It's commonly used in various forms, including capsules, teas, and tinctures, to support mental well-being.

Ashwagandha

For those seeking a more grounding effect, adaptogens like ashwagandha offer valuable support. Ashwagandha is known for its ability to help the body adapt to stress and maintain balance. Its adaptogenic properties can help stabilize mood, increase resilience, and enhance overall emotional resilience.

Lemon Balm

Moreover, lemon balm is another herb with calming and uplifting effects. Often used to reduce anxiety and improve mood, lemon balm can be consumed as a tea or used in essential oil form. Its refreshing and soothing qualities make it a popular choice for those looking to enhance emotional well-being and reduce feelings of nervousness.

Incorporating these herbs into daily routines can provide a natural and effective way to support emotional health. Whether through teas, essential oils, or supplements, these herbal allies offer a gentle touch to maintaining emotional balance and well-being.

Chapter 6

Herbs for the Kitchen

Herbs play a vital role in the kitchen, not just for their flavor, but for their versatile uses and health benefits. Incorporating a variety of herbs into your cooking can elevate dishes and contribute to overall wellness.

Basil

Basil is a quintessential herb that can transform any meal. Its sweet, aromatic flavor enhances everything from tomato sauces to salads. Beyond its culinary uses, basil also offers health benefits. It contains essential oils with anti-inflammatory properties that can support digestion and reduce stress. Fresh basil can be added to dishes right before serving to maintain its vibrant flavor.

Rosemary

Rosemary is another kitchen staple that adds a robust, pine-like flavor to dishes. It's particularly excellent with roasted meats and vegetables. Rosemary is rich in antioxidants and has been shown to support cognitive function and digestion. Infusing rosemary into oils or using it as a seasoning can bring both flavor and health benefits to your meals.

Thyme

Thyme, with its earthy and slightly minty taste, is incredibly versatile. It pairs well with soups, stews, and roasted dishes. Thyme has antimicrobial properties, which can help in maintaining a healthy immune system. It also contains compounds that may improve respiratory health, making it a great addition to your cooking, especially during cold and flu season.

Thyme

Mint, with its refreshing and cooling flavor, is perfect for both sweet and savory dishes. It works well in salads, drinks, and desserts. Mint is known for its digestive benefits, helping to soothe an upset stomach and aid in digestion. Its invigorating scent also has mood-boosting properties.

Parsley

Parsley, often overlooked, is more than just a garnish. Its bright, slightly peppery flavor can enhance soups, stews, and salads. Parsley is rich in vitamins A, C, and K, and has been shown to support heart health and reduce inflammation. Incorporating fresh parsley into your meals can provide a nutrient boost and add a burst of freshness.

Using these herbs not only enriches the flavors of your dishes but also provides a range of health benefits. They can transform ordinary meals into extraordinary experiences while contributing to a balanced and healthful diet.

Chapter 7

Herbs for Children

When it comes to caring for children, herbal remedies can be a gentle and effective way to support their health and well-being. However, it's crucial to use these herbs with care and under the guidance of a healthcare professional. Certain herbs are especially suited for children due to their mild nature and beneficial properties.

Chamomile

One such herb is chamomile. Known for its calming effects, chamomile can help soothe a child's upset stomach or aid in relaxation before bedtime. It's often used in a gentle tea, which can be a comforting routine for children who are feeling anxious or having trouble sleeping. Chamomile tea has been appreciated for its mild, apple-like flavor, making it more palatable for kids.

Peppermint

Peppermint is another versatile herb that can be quite beneficial. It's commonly used to relieve digestive issues such as nausea or indigestion. For children, a mild peppermint tea can provide relief from these symptoms, though it's important to use it sparingly and ensure it's not too strong. Peppermint can also be soothing for minor headaches and colds, adding another layer of comfort.

Echinacea

Echinacea is often associated with immune support and can be helpful for children who are frequent sufferers of colds or infections. Echinacea is thought to boost the immune system, helping the body to fight off illnesses more effectively. However, it's important to note that echinacea should be used cautiously and not as a daily supplement but rather as a supportive treatment during illness.

Ginger

Another herb worth mentioning is ginger, which can be particularly useful for easing nausea and promoting better digestion. A mild ginger tea can be soothing and help with various digestive upsets. Ginger also has anti-inflammatory properties, which can be beneficial for children dealing with sore throats or general discomfort.

Lemon balm

Lastly, lemon balm is a gentle herb known for its calming effects, making it ideal for children experiencing stress or anxiety. Lemon balm can be used in teas or as a mild tincture to help promote a sense of calm and improve sleep quality.

When introducing herbs into a child's regimen, always start with a small amount to ensure there are no adverse reactions and consult with a healthcare provider, especially if the child has underlying health conditions or is taking other medications. Using herbs thoughtfully can provide natural support and complement a child's overall health care routine.

BOOK 3: HERBAL TINCTURES

Chapter 8

What are Tinctures? Remedies and Recipes

Tinctures are a popular way to harness the benefits of herbs in a concentrated, liquid form. They're essentially extracts made by soaking herbs in alcohol or another solvent, which draws out the active compounds from the plant material. This method has been used for centuries to preserve the medicinal properties of herbs and make them more accessible for various health applications.

Creating tinctures involves a simple process: herbs are steeped in a solvent, typically alcohol, for several weeks. This extraction process allows the beneficial compounds in the herbs to dissolve into the liquid, which can then be strained and stored. The result is a potent liquid extract that can be used to address a range of health concerns.

Herbal tinctures are valued for their potency and shelf life. They are easier to take than dried herbs, and their concentrated form means a small amount can be quite effective. Tinctures are also versatile; they can be taken alone, mixed into beverages, or even used topically.

For those interested in making their own tinctures, the process is straightforward. One popular recipe is the tincture of echinacea, often used to support the immune system. To make this tincture, you'd start by;

- Place dried echinacea root in a glass jar
- then cover it with alcohol, such as vodka.
- Seal the jar and let it sit in a cool, dark place for about six weeks
- shake it gently every few days.
- After the steeping period, strain out the herb material, and you're left with a concentrated echinacea tincture that can be used to help boost immune function.

Another common tincture is the peppermint tincture, which can help with digestive issues. To prepare this;

- Fill a jar with dried peppermint leaves, pour alcohol over them until they are fully submerged, and seal the jar. Allow it to sit for four to six weeks, shaking occasionally. Once strained, this tincture can be taken to alleviate symptoms of nausea or indigestion.

For a soothing sleep aid, consider a valerian root tincture.
- Place dried valerian root in a jar and cover it with alcohol. After about six weeks of steeping, strain the mixture. This tincture can help promote relaxation and improve sleep quality.

Each tincture has its unique properties and uses, and the right one for you can depend on your specific needs. Crafting these remedies at home not only allows you to tailor them to your preferences but also provides a deeper connection to the herbal tradition. Whether for personal use or to share with others, tinctures offer a convenient and effective way to incorporate the healing power of herbs into daily life.

Chapter 9

Growing Medicinal Plants

Growing medicinal plants is a rewarding and enriching experience, allowing you to connect more deeply with the herbs you use in your tinctures and other remedies. Cultivating these plants can provide a steady supply of fresh ingredients and a greater understanding of their needs and benefits.

Starting a medicinal garden begins with selecting the right plants for your climate and soil. Many herbs are quite hardy and can thrive in a range of conditions, but it's important to choose those that will do well in your specific environment. Common medicinal plants like lavender, chamomile, and peppermint are not only useful but also relatively easy to grow. Lavender prefers a sunny, well-drained spot, while chamomile and peppermint can adapt to a variety of soil types, though peppermint is best grown in containers to prevent it from overtaking other plants.

Planting your herbs involves more than just putting seeds in the ground. It requires an understanding of their growth habits and care requirements. For instance, peppermint thrives in moist, partially shaded areas, and it can spread rapidly, so it's often grown in pots to keep it contained. On the other hand, lavender needs a lot of sunlight and well-drained soil, making it ideal for a sunny garden bed.

Once your herbs are established, harvesting them at the right time is crucial for maximizing their medicinal properties. For most herbs, the best time to harvest is just before the plants start to flower, as this is when their essential oils and active compounds are most concentrated. Regular pruning helps to encourage healthy growth and prevent the plants from becoming too leggy.

When it comes to creating tinctures from your home-grown herbs, the process is straightforward. For instance, if you've grown calendula, you can make a calendula tincture by filling a jar with the dried flower petals and covering them with alcohol. After allowing the mixture to steep for about six weeks, strain it to obtain a potent tincture that can be used for its soothing properties on the skin.

Another example is making a rosemary tincture. Harvest fresh rosemary, chop it up, and place it in a jar. Cover it with alcohol and let it sit in a dark place for a few weeks. This tincture can be used to support memory and concentration or as a general tonic.

Growing your own medicinal plants not only ensures a fresh supply of herbs but also enhances your connection to natural remedies. It's an opportunity to learn more about each plant's unique characteristics and how to best use them for your health and well-being.

Chapter 10

Organic vs. Non-Organic Gardening

When it comes to gardening, the debate between organic and non-organic methods often boils down to personal philosophy as much as practical outcomes. Organic gardening focuses on cultivating plants in harmony with nature. It eschews synthetic chemicals and fertilizers, emphasizing natural soil amendments, compost, and organic pest control methods. Advocates of organic gardening believe that this approach not only results in healthier plants but also enriches the soil, enhances biodiversity, and contributes to the overall health of the ecosystem. By avoiding chemical pesticides and fertilizers, organic gardeners aim to reduce their environmental footprint and promote a more sustainable way of growing food.

On the other hand, non-organic gardening, which often involves conventional farming practices, uses synthetic chemicals to boost plant growth and manage pests. This method can lead to higher yields and faster growth due to the availability of specialized fertilizers and pesticides. However, there are concerns about the long-term impact on soil health and the environment. The use of synthetic chemicals can sometimes lead to soil degradation and water contamination, raising questions about the broader implications for both the environment and human health.

For those venturing into herbal tincture making, choosing between organic and non-organic herbs can influence the final product. Organic herbs are often preferred for tinctures due to their natural cultivation and the absence of chemical residues, which aligns with the holistic philosophy of herbal medicine. Using organic herbs can ensure that your tinctures are as pure and beneficial as possible, tapping into the full spectrum of the plant's medicinal properties.

When it comes to recipes, using organic herbs in tinctures can elevate the quality of the final product. For instance, making a basic herbal tincture involves infusing chopped herbs in alcohol, allowing the active compounds to be extracted. Using organic herbs means you're likely avoiding exposure to potentially harmful pesticides and fertilizers. A simple recipe might call for filling a jar with chopped organic herbs, covering them with a high-proof alcohol like vodka, and letting the mixture sit for several weeks before straining. This method captures the essence of the herbs in a pure and effective form, benefiting from the natural vibrancy of organically grown plants.

Ultimately, the choice between organic and non-organic gardening practices comes down to individual values and goals. Whether you prioritize sustainability and environmental health or are drawn to the efficiency and results of conventional methods, both approaches offer unique benefits.

BOOK 4: TEAS AND INFUSIONS MADE FROM MEDICINAL HERBS

Chapter 11

What are Teas and Infusions? Uses and Recipes

Teas and infusions are cherished traditions in many cultures, each with its own unique flavors, aromas, and medicinal properties. At their core, teas and infusions involve the extraction of beneficial compounds from plant materials. Though often used interchangeably, they do have distinct differences that influence their preparation and use.

Teas, in the traditional sense, usually refer to beverages made from the leaves of the Camellia sinensis plant, such as black, green, oolong, and white teas. These are crafted through varying levels of oxidation and processing, resulting in a spectrum of flavors and strengths. However, the term "tea" has broadened over time to include herbal blends that don't contain actual tea leaves but are instead made from a diverse range of herbs, flowers, fruits, and spices.

Infusions, on the other hand, are more specifically about steeping plant materials in hot water to extract their essence. This process can involve a variety of herbs, each with its own set of beneficial properties. The term "infusion" often refers to a more prolonged steeping process compared to teas, where the goal is to extract the full range of medicinal compounds from the herbs.

Both teas and infusions offer a soothing way to enjoy the health benefits of herbs. They can be tailored to address various needs, from relaxation to digestion and immune support. For example, a calming tea might feature chamomile and lavender, while a digestive infusion might include peppermint and ginger. These herbal beverages not only provide comfort but also support well-being in gentle and effective ways.

When crafting teas and infusions, the preparation process is straightforward but can be adapted to suit specific needs. To make a basic herbal tea, you start by boiling water and pouring it over a handful of dried or fresh herbs. The steeping time can vary depending on the herb and the desired strength. For example, a mint tea might steep for just a few minutes to deliver a fresh, invigorating flavor, while a more robust blend like chai might require a longer steeping time to fully develop its spices.

Infusions, particularly those aimed at extracting the medicinal properties of herbs, often benefit from longer steeping times. For instance, to make a ginger infusion, you would slice fresh ginger and steep it in hot water for about 15 to 20 minutes. This extended period allows the water to absorb the full spectrum of ginger's beneficial compounds, resulting in a warming, soothing drink that can aid digestion and boost immunity.

When it comes to recipes, creating your own teas and infusions can be both a rewarding and therapeutic process. Here's a simple recipe for a relaxing herbal infusion:

Relaxing Herbal Infusion
- **Ingredients:** 1 tablespoon dried chamomile flowers, 1 tablespoon dried lavender buds, 1 cup boiling water.
- **Instructions:** Combine the chamomile and lavender in a teapot or heatproof container. Pour boiling water over the herbs and cover. Let it steep for 10 to 15 minutes, then strain into a cup. Enjoy this infusion in the evening to unwind before bed.

For a refreshing tea that's great any time of day:

Refreshing Mint Tea
- **Ingredients**: 1 handful fresh mint leaves, 2 cups boiling water, honey (optional).
- **Instructions:** Gently bruise the mint leaves to release their oils and place them in a teapot or heatproof container. Pour boiling water over the leaves and let it steep for about 5 minutes. Strain the leaves, and if desired, sweeten with a touch of honey. This tea is invigorating and great for a midday pick-me-up.

Teas and infusions are more than just beverages; they are a means to connect with nature's remedies and savor the subtleties of plant medicine. Each cup carries the essence of its ingredients, offering comfort, wellness, and a moment of tranquility. Whether you're sipping a calming infusion before sleep or a zesty tea to kickstart your day, these herbal preparations are a simple yet profound way to nurture both body and mind.

BOOK 5: ESSENTIAL OILS APOTHECARY

Chapter 12

What are Essential Oils? Uses and Recipes

Essential oils are concentrated extracts derived from the aromatic compounds of plants. These oils capture the essence of the plant, encapsulating its unique fragrance, flavor, and therapeutic properties. The process of creating essential oils typically involves steam distillation or cold pressing, methods that preserve the potent qualities of the plant material. Each essential oil holds a distinctive profile and can offer a variety of benefits, making them a versatile addition to personal care routines, household cleaning, and even culinary adventures.

The uses of essential oils are as diverse as the plants from which they come. In aromatherapy, essential oils are commonly used to promote emotional and physical well-being. Lavender, for instance, is renowned for its calming properties and is often employed to alleviate stress, improve sleep, and enhance relaxation. Peppermint oil, with its invigorating aroma, can help refresh the mind and ease headaches. Essential oils like tea tree and eucalyptus are celebrated for their antibacterial and antiviral qualities, making them popular choices for supporting respiratory health and maintaining a clean environment.

Beyond their aromatic benefits, essential oils can also be integrated into daily routines through various applications. They are frequently added to skincare products, where their properties can address specific concerns such as dryness, acne, or signs of aging. For example, rosehip oil, known for its regenerative qualities, is a valuable addition to anti-aging serums. Essential oils can also be included in hair care routines to promote healthy scalp conditions and shine.

In the kitchen, essential oils can be used to enhance flavors in cooking and baking. However, due to their potency, they should be used sparingly. A drop of lemon or peppermint oil can provide a burst of flavor that's far more intense than fresh or dried herbs. Always ensure the essential oils used in food preparation are safe for consumption and intended for culinary use.

Creating your own blends and recipes with essential oils allows for a personalized touch. For a relaxing evening, you might prepare a soothing bath blend. Combine a few drops of lavender essential oil with a carrier oil, such as coconut or almond oil, and mix it into your bathwater. This blend can create a tranquil, aromatic experience that helps ease tension and promotes restful sleep.

Another simple yet effective recipe is for a homemade facial toner. Combine 1 tablespoon of witch hazel with 5 drops of tea tree oil and 5 drops of lavender oil. Mix these ingredients and apply to your face with a cotton pad. This toner can help balance the skin, manage acne, and soothe irritation.

For those looking to freshen up their living spaces naturally, a DIY room spray is a great option. Mix 10 drops of eucalyptus essential oil with 2 tablespoons of vodka or rubbing alcohol and 2 cups of water in a spray bottle. Shake well before use and spray around your home to invigorate the air with a crisp, clean scent.

Essential oils offer a wealth of benefits and applications, making them a valuable addition to many aspects of life. By incorporating these oils thoughtfully into your daily routine, you can enjoy their therapeutic properties and rich fragrances, enhancing both your well-being and your environment. Whether used in personal care, cleaning, or culinary endeavors, essential oils bring a natural, aromatic touch to modern living.

BOOK 6: NATURAL HERBAL ANTIBIOTICS

Chapter 13

Harvesting & Processing

Harvesting and processing herbs for natural herbal antibiotics is an art that combines timing, technique, and a bit of patience. The process begins with the careful selection of herbs known for their antimicrobial properties. Plants such as garlic, echinacea, and oregano have been celebrated throughout history for their ability to combat infections and support the immune system.

Timing is crucial when it comes to harvesting. Herbs should be picked at their peak to ensure they contain the highest concentration of active compounds. Generally, this means harvesting herbs when they are fully mature but before they begin to wilt or die back. For example, garlic should be harvested when the lower leaves start to brown but before the bulbs become overripe and begin to split. Similarly, echinacea is best gathered when the flowers are in full bloom, ensuring the maximum potency of its medicinal properties.

Processing herbs correctly is equally important to preserve their therapeutic benefits. After harvesting, herbs should be cleaned to remove any dirt or pests. This is done gently, often by rinsing them in cool water and patting them dry with a clean towel. Proper drying is essential as it prevents mold growth and preserves the herbs' potency. Herbs can be air-dried by hanging them in small bundles in a well-ventilated, dry area away from direct sunlight. Alternatively, a dehydrator or an oven set to a low temperature can be used to speed up the drying process. Once dried, herbs should be stored in airtight containers away from light and moisture to maintain their efficacy.

Creating herbal antibiotics from these processed herbs involves a few simple methods. One common technique is making tinctures, which are alcohol-based extracts that concentrate the herbs' active compounds. To prepare a tincture, finely chop the dried herbs and place them in a jar.

Cover the herbs with a high-proof alcohol like vodka and seal the jar tightly. The mixture should sit in a cool, dark place for several weeks, with occasional shaking to help extract the medicinal properties. After this period, strain the liquid through a fine mesh strainer or cheesecloth, and store it in a dark glass bottle. Tinctures can be used in small doses to support immune function and combat infections.

Another effective method is creating herbal infusions or decoctions, which involve simmering herbs in water to extract their active constituents. For instance, a simple herbal infusion can be made by steeping dried echinacea root in boiling water for 10 to 15 minutes. This method is ideal for herbs that are less potent when dried but still offer valuable medicinal properties. Strain the infusion and enjoy it as a tea, which can help boost the immune system.

For those interested in topical applications, herbal salves can be a useful option. To make a basic salve, infuse dried herbs such as calendula or comfrey in a carrier oil like olive oil. Heat the oil and herbs gently in a double boiler for a few hours, then strain the mixture and combine it with beeswax to achieve the desired consistency. This salve can be applied to minor wounds or skin irritations to promote healing.

Harvesting and processing herbs for natural antibiotics not only connects you with traditional practices but also provides a way to enhance your wellness naturally. By carefully selecting, preparing, and utilizing these herbs, you can create potent remedies that support your health and well-being. Whether through tinctures, infusions, or salves, the process transforms humble plants into powerful allies against illness.

Chapter 14

Using Herbs Safely

Using herbs as natural antibiotics can be a powerful way to support your health, but it's crucial to approach this practice with care and knowledge. While herbs offer many benefits, they also require thoughtful use to ensure safety and effectiveness.

First and foremost, it's essential to understand that not all herbs are suitable for everyone. Individuals with specific health conditions or those who are pregnant or breastfeeding should exercise particular caution. For example, while garlic is known for its antibacterial properties, it can interact with blood-thinning medications, potentially increasing the risk of bleeding. Similarly, echinacea, often used to boost the immune system, might not be suitable for people with autoimmune disorders because it stimulates immune function.

Before incorporating any new herb into your regimen, it's wise to consult with a healthcare provider, especially if you have underlying health conditions or are taking prescription medications. They can provide guidance on potential interactions and ensure that the herbs you choose are appropriate for your specific situation.

Dosage is another crucial aspect of using herbal antibiotics safely. Herbs are potent, and their effects can vary based on the form in which they are used—whether as teas, tinctures, or capsules. It's important to follow recommended dosages and not exceed them, as taking too much can lead to adverse effects. For instance, while a standard dose of garlic might be one or two cloves daily, consuming it in excess could cause digestive upset or bad breath. Always start with a lower dose and observe how your body responds before increasing the amount.

Allergies and sensitivities to herbs can also pose risks. It's advisable to perform a patch test or start with a small amount of the herb to ensure you do not have an adverse reaction. For instance, if you're trying a new topical herbal preparation, apply a small amount to a small area of skin first and monitor for any signs of irritation or allergic response.

When it comes to recipes, ensuring that you use herbs safely involves adhering to proper preparation methods and dosages. A common herbal preparation is a tincture, which can be made by infusing dried herbs in high-proof alcohol. Here's a basic recipe for a garlic tincture:

Garlic Tincture Recipe
- Ingredients: 1 cup chopped fresh garlic, 2 cups vodka (high-proof alcohol).
- Instructions: Place the chopped garlic in a clean jar and pour the vodka over it, ensuring the garlic is fully submerged. Seal the jar tightly and store it in a cool, dark place for about 4 to 6 weeks. Shake the jar daily to help extract the garlic's beneficial compounds. After the tincture has steeped, strain it through a fine mesh strainer or cheesecloth into a clean, dark bottle. This tincture can be used in small doses, typically a few drops to a teaspoon, as needed.

For a simple and soothing herbal tea, try making an echinacea infusion:

Echinacea Tea Recipe
- Ingredients: 1 tablespoon dried echinacea root, 2 cups boiling water.
- Instructions: Place the dried echinacea root in a teapot or heatproof container. Pour boiling water over the root and cover. Let it steep for 10 to 15 minutes. Strain the tea and enjoy it while warm. This infusion can be consumed a few times a day to help support immune function.

Using herbs safely also involves being mindful of their quality. Opt for organic or sustainably sourced herbs whenever possible, as they are less likely to contain harmful pesticides or contaminants. Store your herbs in a cool, dark place to maintain their potency and ensure they remain effective.

Ultimately, the key to using herbs safely is to educate yourself about their properties, consult with healthcare professionals when needed, and use them thoughtfully and responsibly. With proper knowledge and precautions, herbs can be a valuable part of a holistic approach to health, providing natural support and enhancing your well-being.

CONCLUSION

Navigating the world of natural healing through herbal remedies, essential oils, infusions, tinctures, and antibiotics offers a profound journey into the art of holistic wellness. Throughout this guide, we've explored a rich tapestry of knowledge designed to empower you with practical skills and insights for enhancing your health naturally.

Herbal apothecary practices form the cornerstone of this exploration. Understanding how medicinal plants work and the foundational principles of herbal remedies allows you to tap into the healing potential of nature. By delving into the intricacies of how these plants interact with the body, we gain a deeper appreciation for their therapeutic roles and learn to harness their benefits effectively.

Our journey then took us through a comprehensive catalog of herbs, each with its unique properties and applications. From those that support digestive health to herbs that soothe the skin, uplift the spirit, enhance culinary experiences, and cater to the needs of children, this section highlighted the versatility of herbs in daily life. The knowledge of these specific herbs equips you with the tools to address a variety of health concerns and integrate herbal solutions seamlessly into your lifestyle.

The focus on herbal tinctures introduced us to a method of extraction that captures the potent essence of medicinal plants. Understanding what tinctures are, how to make them, and how to cultivate the plants necessary for their creation opens up a new realm of self-sufficiency and personalized health care. We also examined the distinction between organic and non-organic gardening, underscoring the importance of growing practices in ensuring the purity and potency of your herbal preparations.

Teas and infusions provided another avenue for experiencing the benefits of herbs. These simple yet effective preparations offer an accessible way to enjoy the healing properties of plants, whether through a calming tea before bed or a revitalizing infusion during the day. Learning the basics of these beverages, along with practical recipes, allows you to incorporate them into your wellness routine effortlessly.

Essential oils emerged as a powerful component of natural healing, offering a sensory-rich experience through their aromatic and therapeutic properties. By understanding what essential oils are, their diverse uses, and how to make your own blends, you gain a valuable addition to your apothecary. These oils can enhance your physical and emotional well-being, adding depth to your holistic approach to health.

The section on natural herbal antibiotics emphasized the importance of proper harvesting and processing techniques to ensure the effectiveness and safety of herbal remedies. We learned how to handle herbs with care, from collecting them at the optimal time to processing them in ways that preserve their beneficial properties. This careful approach helps maintain the integrity of the herbs, ensuring they deliver their full therapeutic potential.

Safety remains a critical aspect of using herbs. Understanding how to use them responsibly, being aware of potential interactions, and starting with appropriate dosages are essential practices. This guide has equipped you with the knowledge to integrate herbs safely into your life, ensuring that their use is both beneficial and free from adverse effects.

The journey through this book highlights the richness of nature's pharmacy and the empowering ability to take charge of your own health. The practical advice and recipes provided throughout offer a solid foundation for exploring herbal remedies and incorporating them into your daily life. Whether you're creating tinctures, blending essential oils, or brewing herbal teas, the knowledge gained here serves as a stepping stone toward a more natural and balanced approach to wellness.

Embracing these practices not only supports your health but also fosters a deeper connection with the natural world. By cultivating and utilizing healing herbs, you participate in a tradition of self-care that has been cherished across cultures and generations. This holistic approach to health empowers you to live with vitality, supported by the gifts of nature and the wisdom of herbal traditions.